Methylene Blue

From Lab to Life

Alexander Leon

TABLE OF CONTENT

Disclaimer

This book's content is meant primarily for general informational purposes; it should not be used as a substitute for expert medical advice, diagnosis, or treatment. It is not a replacement for expert medical advice from a healthcare provider. A doctor or other trained healthcare practitioner should always be consulted before making any decisions pertaining to your health. The material presented in this book is accurate, up to date, and full, but the author and publisher make no claims or guarantees on this matter. In addition, the publisher and author disclaim any liability for any harm resulting from or related to the use of this book.

INTRODUCTION

Overview of "Methylene Blue: From Lab to Life.

"Methylene Blue: From Lab to Life" is an in-depth investigation that reveals the fascinating path of an extraordinary substance, Methylene Blue, from its beginnings in the lab to its many uses in practical situations. This essay aims to clarify the revolutionary development of Methylene Blue, highlighting its importance and effects on several facets of existence.

The article explores the history of Methylene Blue in the context of laboratories in the first section. It gives historical background, describing the conditions surrounding its synthesis and the trailblazing scientists who worked on its development. This section lays the groundwork for understanding how the chemical evolved from a curiosity in the lab to a material with broad applications.

The features of Methylene Blue, both chemically and visually, are examined in the second part, "A Spectrum of Color and Chemistry". The compound's characteristic blue color and unique qualities are emphasized, highlighting both its aesthetic appeal and the scientific elements that support its adaptability. The foundation for comprehending why Methylene Blue has attracted scientific interest is laid forth in this section.

The essay explores Methylene Blue's entry into the medical sector as it moves into the real world. It highlights the compound's early use for its antibacterial qualities and explores how it moved from the laboratory to the medical field. The article also discusses Methylene Blue's medicinal use in the treatment of diseases like methemoglobinemia, demonstrating how it has grown to be an important tool in the medical toolbox.

In the "*Neurological Significance*" section, the compound's effects on the nervous system are the main topic of investigation. It describes how Methylene Blue may be used to treat neurological conditions including Parkinson's and Alzheimer's. Promising advancements and ongoing research projects highlight the compound's importance in the field of neurology even further.

After that, the topic expands to include "Beyond Medicine: Environmental and Industrial Applications." The contributions of Methylene Blue outside of the medical sector are explained in this section. These include its use in a wide range of industrial processes and as an indicator dye in environmental research. It highlights how versatile and adaptable the chemical is in a variety of scientific fields.

In the "*Challenges and Future Prospects*" section, the article addresses issues related to Methylene Blue as the story progresses. It addresses potential negative repercussions and environmental issues, offering a fair-minded viewpoint. The part also highlights the dynamic character of scientific inquiry by talking about future directions and potential new applications in addition to current research activities.

In the last part, "*Conclusion*," the paper provides an overview of Methylene Blue's amazing voyage. It considers the compound's revolutionary journey, highlighting its significance as evidence of the dynamic relationship between scientific advancement and the wider society. The essay ends with a critical analysis of the relevance of Methylene Blue as a drug that has evolved from its laboratory roots to become a substance that enhances life and has a wide range of uses.

Thesis statement: Exploring the transformative journey of Methylene Blue from laboratory origins to diverse real-world applications.

The central idea of "Methylene Blue: From Lab to Life" is to examine the compound's revolutionary journey, following its development from laboratory beginnings to a variety of real-world uses. A historical examination of Methylene Blue's laboratory beginnings sets the stage for this adventure. The article explores the historical background of Methylene Blue's synthesis and how it came to be throughout its early phases of scientific investigation. Pioneering scientists were vital in bringing this chemical to life in the laboratory's controlled environment because of their curiosity and experimentation.

The article's emphasis moves from the laboratory environment to the physical and chemical properties that characterize Methylene Blue. The compound's unique characteristics and characteristic blue color play a crucial role in comprehending its flexibility. This section lays the groundwork for Methylene Blue's wider applicability outside of the controlled laboratory setting and explains why it has attracted attention from the scientific community.

As Methylene Blue leaves the laboratory and has a big influence on medicine, the story continues to develop. The development of the chemical from a simple laboratory curiosity to a medicinal miracle is examined in this article. The practical uses that sprang from its laboratory roots are highlighted by its early employment as an antiseptic and its medicinal significance in treating illnesses like methemoglobinemia. Methylene Blue's voyage transforms into a real contribution to medical procedures in addition to a scientific investigation.

The investigation continues into the neurological domain, where Methylene Blue indicates its possible utility in treating nervous system diseases. The compound's dynamic significance in neurology is highlighted by ongoing research and exciting advancements, which adds another dimension to its revolutionary journey outside the laboratory.

The article expands its viewpoint by presenting the uses of Methylene Blue in "Beyond Medicine: Environmental and Industrial Applications." Here, the compound's adaptability is demonstrated by its use in several industrial processes and as an indicator dye in environmental science. The variety of uses for Methylene Blue highlights how its journey has taken it well beyond the confines of the laboratory.

The article addresses possible side effects and environmental issues while navigating the difficulties posed by Methylene Blue. The optimism expressed in the "Future Prospects" section is not overshadowed by the examination of the obstacles. Current research endeavors and the possibility of novel applications highlight the compound's dynamic characteristics and its ongoing significance in the ever-changing field of scientific discovery.

The article's conclusion outlines Methylene Blue's remarkable journey, summarizing how it went from being a material created in a lab to having a wide range of practical uses. It considers the compound's value as a witness to the dynamic interaction between scientific advancement and its effects on society at large, in addition to its significance as a scientific curiosity. The investigation of Methylene Blue develops into a story that goes beyond the walls of the lab, demonstrating the compound's ongoing significance in improving and enriching a variety of aspects of life.

CHAPTER I

Origins in the Lab

For more than a century, methylene blue has been utilized as a dye, medicine, and scientific instrument. The German scientist Heinrich Caro created it for the first time in the late 1800s, which is when it all began. However, until the early 20th century, its use in biological systems was not investigated.

American scientist Richard Kuhn carried out one of the first investigations into the effects of methylene blue on living things in the 1930s. While researching how yeast cells metabolize amino acids, Kuhn found that the enzyme that turns tyrosine into dopamine might be inhibited by methylene blue. Following this finding, more research was done to see whether the substance may have an impact on respiration, photosynthesis, and mitosis, among other biological functions.

Researchers kept delving into the characteristics of methylene blue during the ensuing decades and discovered that it was useful in a variety of contexts. For instance, it has been demonstrated to possess antimalarial properties against the malaria-causing organism Plasmodium falciparum. Additionally, it had antiviral and antibacterial qualities, which made it helpful in treating illnesses brought on by bacteria and viruses including herpes simplex virus and Streptococcus pneumoniae.

The potential therapeutic use of methylene blue extended beyond viral disorders. Research findings indicate that this substance possesses anti-inflammatory properties that may mitigate the effects of oxidative stress and tissue damage in situations such as neurological illnesses and arthritis. It has shown promise in the treatment of cancer, especially in photodynamic therapy, in which it preferentially accumulates in tumor cells and, when exposed to light, creates reactive oxygen species that ultimately destroy the tumor cells.

Methylene blue is a useful tool in medicine, scientific study, and diagnostics because of its flexibility. Because of its well-established safety profile and variety of modes of action, it is still routinely utilized today in a wide range of settings, from clinical trials to fundamental research investigations.

Historical context of Methylene Blue's synthesis

German scientist Heinrich Caro, who was employed at Ludwigshafen, Germany's BASF (Badische Anilin- und Soda-Fabrik) chemical business, created methylene blue for the first time in 1876. Methylene blue's synthesis was a noteworthy accomplishment as it was the first coal tar dye to be created artificially as opposed to being taken from plants or animals.

It was long known that coal tar, a byproduct of the gasification of coal, included a range of colorful compounds, but the process of isolating and purifying these chemicals proved to be difficult. Caro created a procedure that included treating the coal tar with sulfuric acid, neutralizing the resultant solution with sodium hydroxide, and then extracting and purifying the colors from the tar. Caro and his colleagues identified and described methylene blue, one of the color mixtures produced by this technique.

A significant development in the field of organic chemistry was made possible by Caro's synthesis of methylene blue, which showed that complex organic compounds could be produced chemically rather than by extraction from natural sources. This accomplishment opened the door for the creation of several additional synthetic colors and medications as well as the advancement of contemporary industrial chemistry.

Plants and animals were the main sources of dyes during the period, and extracting and processing them was frequently costly, time-consuming, and uneven. Larger quantities of colors may be manufactured more swiftly and reliably thanks to the more dependable and affordable option offered by synthesizing dyes from coal tar. This in turn made it possible for dyes to be widely used in printing, textiles, and other industries.

In the textile business, methylene blue has emerged as a significant dye, especially in the manufacturing of cotton and silk garments. In biomedical research, it was also employed as a histological stain to aid in the microscopic examination of the composition and characteristics of cells and tissues. Furthermore, methylene blue contributed to the advancement of contemporary medicine by acting as a model for several medications that are now used to treat a variety of illnesses, such as rheumatoid arthritis, malaria, and some forms of cancer.

All things considered, the creation of methylene blue marks a significant turning point in the history of organic chemistry and shows how human creativity can produce novel materials and cutting-edge technologies that can change the world.

Scientists involved in its creation

Many scientists and researchers have contributed to the discovery and development of methylene blue. Here are a few of the important players:

The invention and synthesis of methylene blue are attributed to Heinrich Caro, a German chemist who worked for the Badische Anilin- und Soda-Fabrik (BASF) in 1876. He created a process for removing and cleaning colors from coal tar, which helped him isolate and identify methylene blue.

2. Eugen Bamberger: a German chemist who worked with Caro at BSF, Bamberger added yield and purity of methylene blue by optimizing the production process. In 1877, Caro and Bamberger jointly submitted a

patent application for the manufacturing of methylene blue.

Carl Liebmann was a German scientist who worked at the University of Berlin. He studied the structural makeup of methylene blue and found that it had the chemical formula $c16h18n3s$. He also investigated its characteristics and behavior, which contributed to proving that it was appropriate for a range of uses.

4. Julius Stieglitz: An Austrian chemist at the University of Vienna, Steglitz carried out a great deal of study on the composition and characteristics of methylene blue in the late 1800s. His research paved the way for the creation of related substances and uses.

Paul Ehrlich, a German physician and chemist who was awarded the Nobel Prize in Physiology or Medicine in 1908, was among the pioneering scientists to acknowledge the medicinal potential of methylene blue. His research opened the door for the use of methylene blue in medicine. He tested the drug's potential for treating several illnesses, such as syphilis and malaria.

6. Ernest Fourneau: a French chemist at the Pasteur Institute in Paris, Fourneau played a key role in creating techniques for producing methylene blue on a large scale during World War I. His work helped guarantee a steady supply of the dye for use in military applications, including communication and camouflage.

7. Louis Goodman: a mid-20th-century American chemist, Goodman worked at the National Bureau of Standards, which is now known as the National Institute of Standards and Technology. Goodman

studied the chemical and physical characteristics of methylene blue. His efforts were directed at enhancing the precision of analytical methods and creating guidelines for the manufacturing and application of methylene blue.

These people have made a substantial contribution to our comprehension and application of methylene blue, along with several others. Their discoveries, inventions, and developments have influenced this compound's history and range of uses.

Significance of its emergence as a dye

The introduction of methylene blue as a dye had profound effects on some industries, such as:

1. Textile Industry: The introduction of methylene blue, an inexpensive, widely available, and very effective dye for dyeing cotton, silk, and wool fibers, completely transformed the textile industry. It took the role of conventional natural dyes like madder and indigo, which were costly, labor-intensive to make, and prone to fading.

2. Art & Design: Because of its vivid, deep blue hue, methylene blue is a preferred option for painters, designers, and crafters. It was widely used to paint, print, and dye textiles for apparel, furniture, and artwork.

3. Biomedical Research: Methylene blue was a useful tool in biomedical research because of its capacity to attach to proteins and nucleic acids. It was used in the study of cellular metabolism, DNA sequencing, and protein structures, leading to important breakthroughs in our comprehension of biological systems.

4. Clinical Diagnosis and Treatment: Methylene blue has been used as a therapeutic drug and diagnostic tool in clinical settings. It was used to treat severe instances of malaria, identify urinary tract infections, and diagnose cyanide poisoning.

5. Food and Cosmetics Industry: To improve the look and appeal of food goods like ice cream and confectionery, methylene blue was added. Due to the rich blue hue, it was also utilized in cosmetics such as lipstick and eye shadow.

6. Environmental Monitoring: By using methylene blue as a tracer dye, scientists were able to monitor pollution, sediment movement, and water flow in rivers, lakes, and seas.

7. Materials Science: Due to methylene blue's special optical and electrical characteristics, it may be used to create cutting-edge materials including polymers, nanoparticles, and solar cells.

8. Photojournalism: Because methylene blue can quickly and reliably generate high-quality photos in challenging circumstances, photojournalists utilized it to develop their shots in the field during World War II.

9. Educational Resources: Methylene blue was used in educational kits and activities to teach students about spectroscopy, chromatography, and acid-base chemistry, among other concepts.

10. Cultural Impact: The unique color of methylene blue has served as an inspiration to poets, singers, and painters, and it has come to represent innovation, inspiration, and metamorphosis.

In conclusion, the discovery of methylene blue as a dye had profound effects on a wide range of academic fields, changing businesses, scientific inquiry, and society at large. Its adaptability, low cost, and vivid color created new avenues for everyday living, scientific research, and creative expression.

Chapter II

A Spectrum of Color and Chemistry

Unique blue hue and visual characteristics

Here are a few methods to characterize methylene blue's distinct blue color and visual attributes:

1. Rich, deep blue hue: Methylene blue is a unique dye or pigment with a rich, deep blue color. Its distinctive blue color is caused by a significant absorption maximum that occurs at around 600 nm in wavelength.

2. High color intensity: Even at low concentrations, methylene blue appears extremely brilliant and vibrant due to its high color intensity. For situations where a strong blue hue is required, this makes it perfect.

3. Low fluorescence: When exposed to UV light, methylene blue exhibits low fluorescence, which implies it does not release much light. It may therefore be applied to situations where the least amount of background fluorescence is required, such as in microscopy and other biological imaging methods.

4. High stability: The chemical and thermal stability of methylene blue is quite high. It is resistant to deterioration over time and can tolerate high temperatures without losing its characteristics or color.

5. Solubility: Methylene blue is easily used in a range of applications since it is soluble in both organic and water-based solvents. It may be readily dissolved in aqueous solutions due to its high water solubility.

6. Versatility: Methylene blue has a wide range of uses, such as cytochemistry, histology, and biomedical imaging. In addition, it may be utilized as a dye for polymers, textiles, and other materials.

7. Non-toxic: Methylene blue is usually regarded as safe to use in a range of applications and non-toxic. It has been safely utilized for some applications, including medical diagnosis and therapy, in both people and animals.

8. Rapid staining: Tissues and cells can be quickly stained with methylene blue, facilitating effective and timely investigation. This is particularly helpful in circumstances when quickness is crucial.

Chemical properties contributing to versatility

The following chemical characteristics of methylene blue help explain its adaptability to a range of applications:

1. pH-dependent solubility: Methylene blue has a 0.5 pKa value, making it somewhat acidic. This indicates that, depending on the pH of the solution, it can exist in both protonated and deprotonated forms. The protonated form is more prevalent at lower pH levels whereas the deprotonated form is more prevalent at higher pH values. Because of this characteristic, methylene blue may be used in a variety of settings, such as neutral, basic, and acidic ones.

2. High ionic strength: Methylene blue may stabilize a variety of ionic species due to its high ionic strength. Because of this characteristic, it may be used in processes like ion exchange and precipitation reactions.

3. Redox characteristics: Methylene blue is capable of participating in redox processes as an acceptor as well as a donor of electrons. Its ability to detect cyanide ions makes it useful in a variety of redox processes.

4. Coordination properties: Methylene blue may form stable complexes by coordinating with metal ions. Because of this feature, it may be applied to chelation treatment and heavy metal detection.

5. Spectral characteristics: The absorption spectra of methylene blue are distinctive, peaking in the yellow-green area at around 600 nm. Because of this characteristic, it may be applied to a variety of spectrum applications, including fluorescence microscopy and visible spectroscopy.

6. Photochemical characteristics: Methylene blue is capable of photoaddition and photocyclization, among other photochemical processes. It may be applied to a variety of tasks, including environmental cleanup and photographic processing, thanks to these interactions.

7. Thermal characteristics: Methylene blue may be used in high-temperature applications due to its high melting and boiling points, which are around 170°C and

380°C, respectively. It can also withstand heat degradation, which enables it to keep its chemical and physical characteristics across a broad temperature range.

8. Substrate specificity: A variety of substrates, including proteins, nucleic acids, carbohydrates, and artificial polymers, can react with methylene blue. Because of this characteristic, it may be used for a variety of tasks, including biomolecular detection and labeling.

An overview of Methylene Blue's unique characteristics

Methylene blue has unique qualities that add to its adaptability and wide range of uses. First of all, its vivid blue color makes it stand out visually and is instantly identifiable. Its use as a dye and indicator in a variety of scientific domains depends on this property.

Methylene blue is known for its redox characteristics, which enable it to both take and provide electrons. This characteristic is utilized in therapeutic settings, where it might function as a mitigating agent for ailments such as methemoglobinemia. Its capacity to traverse biological membranes also helps it in neurological applications, which raises the possibility that it may be used to treat nervous system diseases.

Moreover, Methylene Blue is photoreactive, which means that when it comes into contact with light, it might react chemically.

The compound's versatility beyond conventional applications is demonstrated by the utilization of this characteristic in environmental applications, namely in the degradation of contaminants.

CHAPTER III

Medical Marvel

The transition from laboratory to medical applications

Methylene Blue's shift from laboratory to medical applications entails this compound's adoption and use for a variety of medicinal uses outside of its original laboratory function. In the past, scientists have used Methylene Blue, a synthetic dye with a rich blue hue, to stain biological samples. Nonetheless, due to its special qualities, it may be used in a wider range of medicinal applications.

1. Laboratory Staining: - Methylene Blue first became well-known in labs as a biological stain. To make cells and other biological objects easier to see under a microscope, it was utilized to color them. In the fields of microbiology and histology, this use is essential.

2. Diagnostic Uses: - Methylene Blue has been used in diagnostic imaging. It has helped diagnose several illnesses by being utilized in staining procedures that identify particular cells and structures in clinical samples.

3. Antifungal and Antiseptic Characteristics:
- Methylene blue is appropriate for use in medicine because of its antibacterial and antifungal qualities. It has been applied topically to wounds and infections. Its application has a medicinal component due to its capacity to prevent the development of certain bacteria.

4. Photodynamic Treatment:- The use of Methylene Blue in photodynamic treatment has been investigated recently. Reactive oxygen species are produced when the chemical is activated by light, and these species can specifically kill aberrant cells, including cancerous ones. This application has the potential for treating cancer.

5. Methemoglobinemia Treatment:- An excessive quantity of methemoglobin is created, which lowers the blood's capacity to carry oxygen. Methylene Blue is used in emergency care to treat methemoglobinemia. Methylene Blue aids in the transformation of methemoglobin back into hemoglobin.

6. Neurobiological Effects: - Research indicates that Methylene Blue may be neuroprotective. Its ability to lessen the effects of neurodegenerative illnesses including Parkinson's and Alzheimer's has been studied.

7. Antimalarial Properties:- Studies have also looked at Methylene Blue's antimalarial qualities. It offers a possible therapy option

for malaria as it has demonstrated effectiveness against specific stages of the malaria parasite's life cycle.

The shift from laboratory use to a variety of medicinal applications demonstrates Methylene Blue's adaptability in solving a range of healthcare issues. Because of its qualities, it may be used as a useful tool for therapy, diagnosis, and the treatment of particular medical diseases.

Antiseptic properties and early medical uses of Methylene Blue

Methylene Blue's antiseptic qualities and its early use in medicine:

1. Antibacterial Agent: - Methylene Blue has strong antibacterial characteristics. Early on in its use in medicine, its capacity to stop bacterial development was identified. Because of this characteristic, it was useful for treating wounds and preventing bacterial infections.

2. Malaria Treatment: - Treating malaria was one of the first uses of methylene blue in medicine. Methylene Blue was utilized as a malaria therapy before the invention of contemporary antimalarial medications,

especially in the late 19th and early 20th centuries. It worked well against certain malaria parasite stages.

3. Infections of the Urinary Tract:- In the early stages of treating urinary tract infections (UTIs), methylene blue was used. Because of its antimicrobial qualities, it was helpful in the fight against urinary tract bacterial infections.

The fourth agent is an antifungal one. Methylene Blue has antifungal qualities in addition to its antibacterial ones. Its use in the treatment of fungal diseases during the early days of medicine contributed to its broad-spectrum antibacterial agent properties.

5.Histology Staining:- Histology began to recognize Methylene Blue even before it was used in antiseptic applications. Because of its staining capabilities, scientists and medical experts who are examining tissues under a microscope depend heavily on it. Its wider use in medical diagnostics was made possible by this application.

6. Methemoglobinemia Treatment:- Methemoglobinemia, a disorder marked by high blood levels of methemoglobin, was shown to respond well to Methylene Blue therapy early on. Certain medications or substances may cause hemoglobinemia when they come into contact with them. Methylene Blue aids in the conversion of methemoglobin to functional hemoglobin,

which reinstates the blood's ability to transport oxygen.

7. Topical Antiseptic: - Methylene Blue was administered topically to wounds and injuries to prevent infection because of its antiseptic qualities. Its early use in wound treatment showed how well it promoted healing and decreased the chance of bacterial infection.

8. Surgical Use: - Methylene Blue was first used in surgical settings when it came into usage in medicine. By sterilizing surgical tools and lowering the danger of postoperative infections, its antiseptic qualities were used.

Methylene Blue's antibacterial qualities were a major factor in its widespread usage in medicine. Its early importance in the area of medicine was largely due to its flexibility, ranging from wound care to the treatment of infectious disorders.

Therapeutic role in treating conditions like methemoglobinemia

Methylene Blue's Therapeutic Use in the Treatment of Conditions Like Methemoglobinemia:

1. Action Mechanism: - As a reducing agent, methylene blue's capacity to convert non-functional methemoglobin back into functional hemoglobin underpins its therapeutic use in diseases like

methemoglobinemia. When methemoglobin levels rise abnormally, it becomes methemoglobinemia because it is unable to carry oxygen efficiently.

2. Methemoglobinemia Treatment: The first line of therapy for acquired methemoglobinemia, which is often brought on by exposure to certain medications, chemicals, or poisons, is methylene blue. It helps the blood's ability to transport oxygen be restored by facilitating the conversion of methemoglobin to hemoglobin.

3. Emergency Circumstances: - When methemoglobinemia is severe, Methylene Blue is injected intravenously in emergency treatment. This early action is critical, particularly in cases where tissues are not

receiving enough oxygen due to excessive methemoglobin levels.

4. Rapid Reversal of Symptoms: - Methylene Blue causes methemoglobinemia symptoms, such as cyanosis (bluish coloring of the skin and mucous membranes), to rapidly reverse. It increases oxygenation and provides rapid symptom relief by speeding up the conversion of methemoglobin to hemoglobin.

5. Administration and Dosage: – In a medical environment, Methylene Blue is usually injected intravenously. The patient's weight and the degree of methemoglobinemia will determine the dose. Medical personnel keep a careful eye

on how the patient is responding to their care.

6. Monitoring Oxygen Saturation: - To guarantee the efficacy of the therapy, medical professionals keep an eye on oxygen saturation levels when administering Methylene Blue. Ongoing observation aids in evaluating the patient's reaction and directs further treatments as needed.

Even though Methylene Blue is usually well tolerated, healthcare professionals take into account several considerations before starting therapy, including the patient's medical history, possible medication interactions, and glucose-6-phosphate dehydrogenase (G6PD) deficiency.

8. Pediatric utilize: - Children with methemoglobinemia may also utilize Methylene Blue. Reversing methemoglobinemia-induced symptoms quickly is the treatment's guiding concept, and the dose is modified according to the child's weight.

9. Research and Advancements: - Current investigations examine the use of Methylene Blue in various therapeutic contexts and its possible advantages beyond the management of methemoglobinemia. This involves examining its neuroprotective properties and considering its use in combination treatments for a range of ailments.

Methylene blue plays a vital role in regaining normal hemoglobin function and handling potentially fatal situations, as shown by its therapeutic use in the treatment of disorders such as methemoglobinemia. For methemoglobinemia symptoms to be effectively and quickly reversed, it must be administered as soon as possible.

CHAPTER IV

Neurological Significance

Exploration of Methylene Blue's impact on the nervous system

Examining the Effects of Methylene Blue on the Nervous System:

1. Neuroprotective Properties: - Studies have indicated that Methylene Blue benefits the nervous system. It's worth investigating as a potential therapy for neurodegenerative

illnesses since it could shield neurons from harm and death.

2. Alzheimer's Disease: - Research has looked at the possible application of Methylene Blue in Alzheimer's patients. The substance has demonstrated some potential in lowering tau protein aggregation, which is linked to neurofibrillary tangles in Alzheimer's sufferers' brains.

3. Parkinson's Disease: - Methylene Blue has been researched about Parkinson's disease to assess its ability to reduce oxidative stress and safeguard dopaminergic neurons. These brain neurons' deterioration is a hallmark of Parkinson's disease.

4. Antioxidant Effects: - Methylene Blue neutralizes reactive oxygen species, which can cause cellular damage, by acting as an antioxidant. This antioxidant function is especially important for the brain system, as oxidative stress has been linked to many neurological conditions.

5. Mitochondrial Function: - The effects of Methylene Blue on mitochondrial function have been investigated. Numerous neurological disorders are linked to mitochondrial malfunction, and the potential benefits of Methylene Blue for maintaining mitochondrial health may extend to neuroprotection.

6. Improvement of Cognitive Ability: - According to certain research, Methylene

Blue may improve cognitive function. Improvements in memory and cognitive function are part of this. The intricate processes behind these impacts might entail adjustments to neurotransmitter systems.

7. Potential for Stroke therapy: - Methylene blue has been studied as a possible ischemic stroke therapy. Methylene Blue may help lessen the consequences of stroke-related brain damage by enhancing blood flow and having neuroprotective effects.

8. Nitric Oxide Modulation: - It has been demonstrated that methylene blue affects nitric oxide levels, which are important for neurotransmission. This modification may have consequences for diseases in which dysregulation of nitric oxide is present.

9. Averting Cognitive Deterioration: - Research is still being conducted to see whether Methylene Blue can help avoid the cognitive deterioration that comes with age. It is a fascinating candidate for more research due to its diverse processes, which include antioxidant qualities and possible impacts on protein aggregation.

10. Clinical Trials and Future Directions:- Methylene Blue's safety and effectiveness in treating a range of neurological diseases are still being evaluated in clinical trials. The objective of these studies is to provide more tangible proof of its influence on the neurological system and its possible use as a medicinal agent.

Although research on Methylene Blue's effects on the nervous system is still in its early stages, preliminary findings point to a variety of possible advantages, from neuroprotection to cognitive improvement. Further research and clinical trials will enhance our comprehension of its function in treating neurological conditions.

Potential applications in addressing neurological disorders

Alzheimer's illness:

The possibility of methylene blue in Alzheimer's disease has been studied. According to studies, it could lessen the tau protein's tendency to aggregate and create neurofibrillary tangles in Alzheimer's patients' brains. Its neuroprotective qualities could be advantageous for treatment.

Parkinson's illness:

Because of Methylene Blue's neuroprotective properties, it may be used to treat Parkinson's disease. Studies suggest that it could shield dopaminergic neurons, whose deterioration is linked to Parkinson's disease. Because of its antioxidant qualities, it may be able to lessen the oxidative stress linked to the illness.

Ischemic Concussion:

Preclinical research has demonstrated the possibility of methylene blue as an ischemic stroke therapy. Enhancing blood circulation and exhibiting neuroprotective properties, might potentially mitigate the extent of harm resulting from the absence of blood flow to the brain during a stroke.

Improving Cognitive Function:

Methylene blue may improve memory and other aspects of cognitive function, according to studies. This has consequences for treating neurodegenerative diseases and age-related cognitive decline. These cognitive advantages could be attributed to the compound's capacity to modify neurotransmitter networks.

Neuropathic Pain:

The potential of methylene blue in the treatment of neuropathic pain has been investigated. Because neuropathic pain disorders are complicated, their methods of action, which include effects on nitric oxide and antioxidant characteristics, may be useful in treating them.

Enzyme-Related Disorders:

Methylene Blue has been thought of in mitochondrial illnesses because of its effect

on oxidative stress and mitochondrial function. Because the energy-producing mitochondria frequently malfunction in these conditions, Methylene Blue's supporting function may be advantageous.
Injury to the Brain (TBI):

Regarding traumatic brain damage, methylene blue is a topic of research due to its neuroprotective and anti-inflammatory qualities. It could lessen the chance of brain trauma resulting in subsequent damage.
The disease known as Huntington's

Methylene blue may be able to treat Huntington's disease, according to research. Its potential to defend against oxidative stress and regulate cellular processes may be important in lessening the effects of this inherited neurodegenerative illness.

Conditions Neuroinflammatory:

Methylene Blue's anti-inflammatory qualities could be useful in treating neuroinflammatory diseases. Numerous neurological illnesses are influenced by inflammatory processes, and Methylene Blue's capacity to control these reactions may have therapeutic benefits.

Depressive and Mood Conditions:

Methylene Blue may have antidepressant properties, according to certain research. Due to its impact on serotonin and other neurotransmitter systems, it may be a good option for treating mood disorders.

Sustained investigation and clinical studies are necessary to confirm and enhance the possible uses of Methylene Blue in neurological conditions. Although encouraging, further research is necessary to determine the safety and effectiveness of therapies based on Methylene Blue due to the complexity of these illnesses.

Overview of ongoing research and promising developments

1. Diseases Related to Neurodegeneration: - The use of Methylene Blue in the treatment of neurodegenerative illnesses like Parkinson's and Alzheimer's is probably the subject of ongoing study. Comprehending its mechanisms of action and maximizing doses for therapeutic effectiveness may be the main emphasis.

2. Stroke Treatment: - Studies on Methylene Blue's ability to treat ischemic stroke may still be ongoing. To evaluate its safety and efficacy in humans, this may entail preclinical research, animal testing, or early-phase clinical trials.

3. Cognitive Enhancement:- Further clarification of Methylene Blue's effects on cognitive function may be a promising advance in the field of cognitive enhancement. Clinical trials may investigate its use in disorders linked to cognitive impairment or decline.

4. Neuropathic Pain Management:- The usefulness of Methylene Blue in treating neuropathic pain may be the subject of ongoing study. To ascertain its function in

reducing pain related to nerve injury, this may entail both lab research and clinical trials.

5. Diseases of the Mitochondrion: - Future studies may concentrate on comprehending how Methylene Blue might assist mitochondrial function as well as its possible uses in conditions where mitochondrial malfunction is present.

6. Psychiatric Conditions: - Research on Methylene Blue's antidepressant properties and its uses in mood disorders may still be ongoing. Its effects on the neurotransmitter systems involved in mood regulation may be the subject of future research.

7. Optimizing Treatment Protocols: - Research might focus on improving treatment plans for ailments where Methylene Blue has demonstrated potential. This may entail figuring out the best doses, modes of administration, and possible interactions with additional treatments.

8. Safety and Side Effects: - Ongoing studies are probably aimed at assessing Methylene Blue's safety profile, particularly when it comes to extended or erratic use. For the chemical to have wider medical use, it is essential to comprehend potential adverse effects and confirm the compound's safety in various patient populations.

9. Combination Therapies: - Further study may be conducted to see how well

Methylene Blue works in conjunction with other therapies for different ailments. This strategy can focus on treating several facets of complicated illnesses or have synergistic benefits with current medicines.

10. Pharmacokinetics and Bioavailability:- Methylene Blue's pharmacokinetics and bioavailability may be the subject of ongoing research. To optimize its therapeutic usage, it is important to comprehend the processes by which the substance is absorbed, distributed, metabolized, and excreted by the body.

Checking current scientific literature, clinical trial databases, and updates from respectable medical and research institutes are advised ways to stay up to speed on Methylene Blue research and advances.

CHAPTER V

Beyond Medicine

Environmental applications, including its role as an indicator dye

Methylene Blue's Use in the Environment, Including Its Function as an Indicator Dye:

1. Water Quality Evaluation - When analyzing water quality, methylene blue is frequently employed as an indicator dye. Its color shift can indicate the presence of reducing agents or a water sample's potential for reduction, giving information

about the general quality of the water as well as its ability to support certain biological activities.

2. Oxygen Detection: - Methylene blue can serve as an indication of oxygen present in environmental research. It may be used in studies and field evaluations about oxygen availability in aquatic habitats because of its capacity to change color in response to differences in oxygen levels.

3. Measurement of Redox Potential: - Methylene Blue is used to determine the redox potential of soil and water. It can provide important information for ecological and environmental research by indicating the reducing or oxidizing characteristics of an environment.

4. Soil Analysis: - Methylene Blue is used in soil science to evaluate the qualities of soil. Its use advances knowledge of soil fertility and health by assisting in the determination of soil structure and cation exchange capacity.

5. Evaluation of Microbial Activity: - Environmental sample microbial activity may be detected using Methylene Blue. Studies on the microbiology of soil and wastewater treatment can benefit from the understanding that color changes might represent differences in the metabolic activity of microorganisms.

6. Wastewater Treatment:- Processes for treating wastewater have made use of

Methylene Blue. Its capacity to interact with microbes and organic materials makes it valuable for evaluating the effectiveness of treatment techniques as well as the general caliber of wastewater that has been treated.

7. Aquaculture Studies: - To evaluate water quality parameters, aquaculture research uses Methylene Blue. Its use enables researchers to keep an eye on factors that affect aquatic life, such as oxygen concentrations and the presence of compounds that are harmful to fish health.

8. Dye Tracing in Studies on Groundwater: - Methylene Blue has been utilized as a dye tracer in groundwater research in environmental hydrology. Researchers can learn more about the patterns of

groundwater flow and pinpoint possible sources of pollution by following the dye's path.

9. Bioremediation Monitoring: Methylene Blue can be used to keep an eye on the processes involved in bioremediation. By using it, scientists can monitor microbial activity and evaluate how well biological treatments work to remove contaminants from the environment.

10. Educational Demonstrations: – Methylene Blue is used to illustrate a variety of chemical and environmental concepts in educational contexts. Because of its ability to change color, it's a visually stimulating teaching tool for redox processes, microbiology, and environmental science.

Beyond lab settings, methylene blue serves as an indicator dye that is useful for observing and assessing environmental conditions. Because of its adaptability, researchers and environmental specialists may evaluate and enhance the condition of ecosystems and water resources with the help of this valuable instrument.

Industrial uses showcase versatility beyond

1. Water treatment: To eliminate pollutants and impurities from wastewater and drinking water, methylene blue is employed as an oxidizing and disinfecting agent in water treatment procedures. It is an efficient instrument for water purification since it can eradicate viruses, bacteria, and fungi.

2. Textile industry: A variety of green, blue, and purple hues are produced in this sector by using methylene blue as a dye. Additionally, it is used as a finishing agent to enhance the longevity and colorfastness of textiles.

3. Paper manufacture: To increase the strength and durability of paper products, methylene blue is employed as a sizing agent throughout the paper production process. Higher-quality paper products are produced as a consequence of their assistance in keeping the fibers from disintegrating throughout the production process.

4. Food and beverage industry: Certain foods and beverages employ methylene blue as a preservation and food ingredient. Fruit juices, soft drinks, and bottled water all include it to keep them fresher longer.

5. Pharmaceuticals: Because of its antibacterial qualities, methylene blue has been employed in medicinal applications. It serves as an intermediary in the manufacture of certain medications, such as

anti-inflammatory and antibacterial substances.

6. Biotechnology: The possible application of methylene blue in biotechnology processes like gene therapy and bioconjugation has been studied. It is a good option for delivering therapeutic genes or imaging agents to certain cells or tissues because of its capacity to attach to DNA and other macromolecules.

7. Environmental remediation: The possibility of using methylene blue to remove contaminants from soil and groundwater has been investigated. It can more easily remove organic molecules and heavy metals from the environment by preferentially adhering to them.

8. Cosmetics: Because methylene blue imparts a variety of hues, it is utilized in

cosmetic items including lipsticks, eye shadows, and hair dyes. Because of its anti-inflammatory and antioxidant qualities, it is also utilized in skincare products.

9. Photography: To remove unexposed silver halides from photographic film and paper, methylene blue has been employed as a fixer in photographic processing.

10. Medical diagnostics: To identify cyanide poisoning, methylene blue has been utilized as a diagnostic tool in medical settings. It functions by forming a stable compound that may be detected via spectrophotometry through a reaction with cyanide ions.

These illustrations show the wide variety of sectors and uses for which methylene blue is useful because of its special chemical and physical characteristics.

Highlighting Methylene Blue's impact in diverse fields

The adaptable substance methylene blue has had a profound effect on several industries, including science, technology, and medicine. The following are some areas where methylene blue has had an impact:

1. Medicine

Methemoglobinemia treatment: Methemoglobinemia is a condition where the blood's concentration of methemoglobin rises, depriving the body's tissues of oxygen. Methylene blue is used to treat this disease. By changing methemoglobin back into hemoglobin, methylene blue facilitates the return of oxygen to the bloodstream.

Antimalarial medication: Methylene blue is a medication that has been used to treat malaria, especially Plasmodium falciparum malaria. It functions by disrupting the parasite's energy metabolism, which finally causes it to perish.* Neuroprotection: Studies indicate that methylene blue may have neuroprotective properties, which may aid in the treatment or prevention of neurodegenerative illnesses like Parkinson's and Alzheimer's.

2. Science

Chemical processes: A frequent reagent in chemical reactions, such as the detection of cyanide ions, is methylene blue. Additionally, it can catalyze several processes, increasing their yield and efficiency.* Dye: Methylene blue is a dye that is used in many different fields, such as histology, to stain tissue samples so that scientists may examine cellular structures under a microscope.* Analytical chemistry: By observing how methylene blue's absorption spectrum varies as it binds to specific molecules, such as proteins, carbohydrates, and lipids, one may utilize this technique to identify the presence of specific chemicals.

3. Technology:

Water treatment: To eliminate contaminants and cleanse water, methylene blue is used in water treatment procedures. It can help get rid of smells and cloudiness from water and destroy dangerous pathogens including viruses and bacteria. Papermaking: To improve the strength and brightness of paper products, the papermaking business uses methylene blue. This is achieved by lowering the content of lignin, a naturally occurring polymer that may give the paper a yellow tint and impair its structure. * Food and drink: Methylene blue is occasionally added as a preservative to food and drink to prolong its shelf life by halting the growth of microbes.

4. Agriculture

Regulation of plant growth: It has been demonstrated that methylene blue affects the growth and development of plants, especially in the creation of roots and shoots. * It can also boost agricultural production and have an impact on floral coloration. Crop protection: The use of methylene blue as a possible defense against pests and diseases has been studied. It can deter insects that prey on plants and inhibit the growth of bacteria and fungi that cause plant illnesses.

CHAPTER VI

Challenges and Future Prospects

Addressing challenges associated with Methylene Blue

Although methylene blue has a lot of useful uses, there are several drawbacks to its employment. Among the principal difficulties are:

1. Toxicity: Long-term exposure to low amounts of methylene blue can nonetheless be harmful to one's health. The chemical can be poisonous at large concentrations. To reduce exposure, proper handling, storage, and disposal practices are crucial.

2. Resistance: Misuse or overuse of Methylene Blue can cause germs to become resistant to it, which reduces its efficacy as an antiseptic or disinfectant. This emphasizes how crucial it is to use the substance sparingly and only when essential.

3. Interaction with other drugs: Methylene Blue may combine with several drugs, including antidepressants, to produce serotonin syndrome, which is a potentially fatal illness. When receiving Methylene Blue, patients who are taking these drugs should be thoroughly observed.

4. Allergic reactions: Methylene Blue may cause allergic responses in certain people, which can range from minor skin irritation to life-threatening anaphylaxis. Healthcare professionals need to be on the lookout for allergy symptoms in their patients and treat them appropriately when necessary.

5. Cost: Methylene Blue may be pricey, particularly when used in big quantities. This could restrict its use for non-essential applications or in environments with limited resources.

6. Environmental problems: Because Methylene Blue may build up in soil and streams and possibly harm wildlife, its usage in agriculture and aquaculture raises environmental concerns. Regulations and appropriate disposal techniques are essential for reducing these threats.

7. Adequate regulatory frameworks are necessary to ensure the safe and responsible use of Methylene Blue. Nonetheless, regulatory disparities or discrepancies may occur among nations or areas, creating difficulties for global trade and public health initiatives.

8. Lack of knowledge: A lot of individuals are not aware of the advantages and dangers of Methylene Blue. It is crucial to teach farmers, medical experts, and the general public how to use and handle the substance safely.

9. Limited accessibility: Methylene Blue may not be easily accessible or available in some regions of the world, which makes it difficult to utilize in urgent situations. This problem can be solved in part by strengthening supply chains and distribution networks.

10. Future developments: The need for Methylene Blue may decline if substitutes and new technologies become available. To keep it relevant and successful in a variety of applications, ongoing research and innovation are required.

It will need a coordinated effort from governments, healthcare institutions, business executives, and ordinary users to address these issues. Together, we can make sure that Methylene Blue is used sustainably and safely for many years to come.

Consideration of potential side effects and environmental concerns

Possible Adverse Reactions:

1. Allergic Reactions: Methylene blue allergies can result in symptoms including breathing difficulties, redness, swelling, and itching.

2. Nausea and Vomiting: Methylene blue may induce nausea and vomiting, particularly in cases when large dosages or prolonged exposure are administered.

3. Headache and Dizziness: Methylene blue may result in headaches and, in certain situations, severe dizziness.

4. Skin Discoloration: Methylene blue usage over an extended period might result in skin discoloration, especially in sun-exposed regions.

5. Blood diseases: Methylene blue can impact the synthesis of platelets, white blood cells, and red blood cells, which can result in blood diseases such as thrombocytopenia, leukopenia, and anemia.

6. Liver Damage: Extended exposure to methylene blue can harm the liver, especially in those who already have liver problems.

7. Kidney Issues: Methylene blue can build up in the kidneys and harm them, especially in those who already have kidney issues.

Environmental Issues:

1. Water Pollution: Fish and other marine life are especially vulnerable to the harmful effects of methylene blue, which can taint water supplies.

2. Soil Pollution: In regions where methylene blue is widely used in agriculture, it can also pollute soil and hinder plant development.

3. Bioaccumulation: Methylene blue may build up in both human and animal systems, especially in fatty tissues, where it can have long-term negative consequences on health.

4. Resistance: Excessive usage of methylene blue might result in the emergence of germs resistant to it, which can lessen its efficacy as an antiseptic and disinfectant.

5. Disposal: If methylene blue is disposed of improperly, it may contaminate the environment, especially if it seeps into soil or rivers.

Consideration of potential side effects and environmental concerns

Methylene blue can be used in a variety of applications, but it's crucial to carefully assess any potential negative consequences and environmental issues. Here are some things to think about:

1. Hazards to Human Health: a. Allergic responses: In certain people, methylene blue can trigger allergic responses, which can vary in severity from less severe symptoms

like swelling, redness, and itching to more serious ones like anaphylaxis.

b. Respiratory Problems: Breathing in large amounts of methylene blue vapor can lead to lung damage, asthma attacks, and bronchitis. Over time, lung problems may also arise from prolonged exposure to lower doses.

c. Eye irritation: Prolonged exposure to methylene blue might result in visual issues as well as inflammation of the eyes.

d. Skin Sensitivity: Direct contact with methylene blue can lead to burns, rashes, or skin irritation. It can also induce skin sensitivity.

e. Gastrointestinal Problems: Consuming methylene blue may result in diarrhea, vomiting, nausea, and upset stomach.

2. Environmental Issues: a. Water Pollution: Methylene blue has the potential to poison water supplies, endangering ecosystems and aquatic life. It can linger in water systems for long periods and is not readily broken down.

b. Soil Pollution: Methylene blue can pollute soil, which may hinder plant development and harm ecosystems over time.

c. Air Pollution: Methylene blue emissions into the atmosphere have the potential to aggravate respiratory conditions and other health concerns in the populations they may affect.

d. Accumulation in Organisms: When methylene blue builds up in the tissues of living things, it may be harmful to people and wildlife alike who eat polluted food or drink.

3. Safe Handling and Disposal: Methylene blue must be handled carefully and disposed of appropriately to reduce dangers. This includes keeping it out of direct sunlight, away from heat sources and other choking dangers, and disposing of it according to approved procedures.

4. Alternatives: It's vital to think about safer and less environmentally damaging options before using methylene blue. Alternatives like ozone or UV light disinfection, for instance, maybe more efficient and ecologically beneficial when it comes to water treatment.

5. Risk Assessment and Management: Before the use of methylene blue in any application, a comprehensive risk assessment must be carried out. This should involve determining the best exposure

routes, doses, and times, as well as putting precautions in place to reduce risks and handle any negative consequences.

6. Regulatory Compliance: When using, managing, and disposing of methylene blue, users must make sure they comply with all applicable laws and guidelines. This covers adhering to worker safety regulations, safeguarding the environment, and fulfilling labeling specifications.

7. Public Education and Training: Methylene blue handlers have to be properly trained in the safe use, handling, and disposal of the chemical. The general public should also be informed on the advantages and possible hazards of methylene blue, as well as how to handle and dispose of it securely.

8. Emergency Response Plan: If methylene blue is unintentionally released or spilled, an emergency response plan has to be created and put into action. Procedures for treating those who have been exposed, cleaning up spills, and reducing the impact on the environment should all be outlined in this strategy.

9. Monitoring and Testing: To make sure that safety regulations are being followed and to spot any possible dangers or adverse effects, routine monitoring and testing of the levels of methylene blue in water, soil, and air should be carried out.

10. Constant Review and Update: To make sure that methylene blue continues to be a safe and useful solution for a range of applications, the risks and advantages of the substance should be constantly evaluated

and updated as new information becomes available.

Methylene blue has advantages, but there are also drawbacks. These may be avoided by carefully weighing these considerations and implementing the necessary precautions to reduce hazards.

Looking ahead to ongoing research and future applications

Methylene blue is being researched in the following areas for potential future uses:

1. Cancer treatment: Methylene blue is being investigated for use in photodynamic

therapy (PDT) as a photosensitizer. PDT includes the injection of a photosensitizer, which is activated by exposure to a certain wavelength of light and causes the cancer cells to be destroyed. Early clinical trials have demonstrated the potential of methylene blue as a photosensitizer for photodynamic therapy (PDT) in the treatment of several cancer types, such as skin, lung, and breast malignancies.

2. Neurodegenerative illnesses: Possible treatments for neurodegenerative illnesses including Alzheimer's, Parkinson's, and Huntington's disease have been explored, including methylene blue. According to studies, methylene blue may have neuroprotective properties and aid in lowering inflammation and oxidative stress in the brain.

3. Treatment for malaria: Methylene blue has been researched as a possible remedy for malaria, especially for strains that are not amenable to conventional therapies. Malaria parasite development has been demonstrated to be inhibited by methylene blue, which may be helpful when used in conjunction with other medications to treat resistant strains of the illness.

4. Wound healing: Methylene blue has been studied as a topical wound therapy, especially for infected or slowly healing wounds. According to studies, methylene blue may speed up the healing of wounds by boosting blood flow and lowering the development of germs.

5. Dental applications: Periodontitis and oral thrush are two dental disorders for which methylene blue has been investigated

as a possible therapy. It may be helpful as a mouthwash or topical therapy since it has been demonstrated to reduce the growth of the bacteria and fungi that cause these illnesses.

6. Anti-aging: Because of its capacity to lower oxidative stress and scavenge free radicals, methylene blue has been marketed as an anti-aging agent. Although there isn't much scientific proof to back up its usage for this purpose, some studies indicate that it could improve the look of wrinkles and skin tone.

7. Veterinary medicine: Several ailments, including bacterial, fungal, and parasitic diseases, have been treated using methylene blue in veterinary medicine. Additionally, it has been employed as a diagnostic

technique to find certain medical issues in animals.

Conclusion

Summary of Methylene Blue's transformative journey

The synthetic dye methylene blue has come a long way from its original discovery to its current use in a wide range of industries. This is a quick rundown of its journey:

1. *Discovery:* German scientist Heinrich Caro produced methylene blue for the first time in 1876. It was first applied as a dye for paper and textiles.

2. *Early medical applications:* Methylene blue was first applied to treat a variety of ailments in the late 1800s, such as malaria, typhoid fever, and cyanide poisoning.

3. Antibacterial qualities: Methylene blue was used to treat bacterial diseases, including septicemia and urinary tract infections when researchers identified its antibacterial qualities in the middle of the 20th century.

4. Psychiatric applications: Methylene blue was employed in psychiatry to treat anxiety, depression, and other mental health issues throughout the 1950s and 1960s. It was thought to function by raising certain neurotransmitter levels in the brain.

5. Cancer therapy: Methylene blue has recently been researched as a possible treatment for lung, breast, and colon cancers, among other cancer types. It has been demonstrated to cause apoptosis, or cell death, and to impede the proliferation of cancer cells.

6. Neuroprotection: Research on the possible neuroprotective properties of methylene blue has revealed that it may help fend against neurodegenerative illnesses including Alzheimer's, Parkinson's, and Huntington's diseases.

7. Energy applications: Because methylene blue can transmit electrons and absorb light, it has been investigated as a possible component of solar cells and batteries.

8. Environmental applications: Methylene blue has been looked into as a possible solution for cleaning up oil spills and has been used to extract heavy metals and other contaminants from wastewater.

Considering its importance as a substance with a variety of practical uses.

Methylene blue is a very adaptable substance that has several important real-world uses in a variety of sectors. Because of its special qualities, it is a vital instrument in many scientific disciplines, such as biology, chemistry, energy, and environmental research. The following are some thoughts about the relevance of methylene blue as a substance with a variety of practical uses:

1. Biomedical Applications: Malaria, cancer, and neurological diseases are just a few of the illnesses for which methylene blue has proven to be extremely helpful in diagnosis and treatment. It is an important tool in genetic engineering and molecular biology due to its capacity to attach to proteins and DNA. Furthermore, it is a good option for the development of novel medications and treatments due to its antibacterial and anticancer qualities.

2. Chemical Synthesis: Methylene blue finds extensive application as a catalyst in chemical synthesis, especially in the manufacturing of agrochemicals, medicines, and materials for energy conversion and storage. Because of its capacity to promote chemical reactions and create complexes with metal ions, it is an essential part of several industrial processes.

3. Energy Applications: Research has been done on methylene blue as a possible material for energy conversion and storage, especially in solar cells and batteries. Because of its capacity to both transport electrons and absorb light, it is a viable option for increasing the efficiency of renewable energy technology. Its availability and inexpensive cost in comparison to conventional materials also make it a desirable choice for widespread use.

4. Environmental Science: By using methylene blue as a tracer, scientists can monitor the migration and eventual fate of contaminants in soil and water. It's a useful tool for cleaning up polluted areas and studying how pollutants behave in the environment because of its capacity to bind to heavy metals and other contaminants.

5. Food Industry: Methylene blue is used as a preservative and food additive, especially in the manufacturing of dairy and meat products. Its antibacterial qualities contribute to food safety and quality by extending shelf life and preventing spoiling.

6. Textile business: A variety of hues and tones for fabrics have been achieved by the use of methylene blue as a dye in this business. It is a common option for making strong, colorfast textiles because of its capacity to bond to cotton and other natural fibers.

Closing thoughts on the dynamic interplay between science and the broader world.

The dynamic and varied relationship that exists between research and the outside world has important implications for both the scientific community and society at large. Here are my final thoughts on the matter:

1. Science and society are closely related to one another. Although science and technology have the potential to greatly advance humanity, some risks and unknowns need to be appropriately considered. Our choices on the application of scientific and technical advances have ethical implications that need to be carefully thought out.

2. Scientific literacy is essential: We need to be scientifically educated to make informed decisions about issues that affect our lives as citizens. Critical evaluation of the evidence is vital, as is an understanding of the implications of scientific and technical breakthroughs.

3. It is imperative that scientists and non-scientists work together: Science nowadays requires collaboration between experts from many domains and interested persons from a variety of socioeconomic backgrounds; it is no longer a solitary undertaking. By working together, we may develop solutions that satisfy societal objectives and goals.

4. Communication is crucial: Effective communication between scientists, decision-makers, and the general public is necessary to build trust and encourage discussion on scientific subjects. We need to find a way to communicate complex scientific concepts in plain language without sacrificing accuracy or nuance.

5. Ethics must be included in scientific research: As scientists, it is our responsibility to carry out our work in an ethical manner, taking into account any potential consequences of our conclusions. This means having open discussions about the study's ethical ramifications and considering a variety of points of view when making decisions.

6. Reputable data and professional counsel ought to inform choices about science and technology policy: Decisions about science and technology policy should be supported by substantial evidence. Policymakers must be willing to support scientific research and heed scientific advice when making decisions that will affect society.

7. Society must be prepared to adapt to new scientific knowledge: As science develops and new understandings of the world are obtained, society must be prepared to change and advance. This means acknowledging the dangers and limitations associated with new ideas and technical developments while also embracing them.

8. Science education should encourage critical thinking and curiosity: Apart from imparting critical thinking skills to students so they can evaluate the data and draw well-informed conclusions, science education ought to encourage in them a sense of awe and enthusiasm for the natural world.

9. Science and culture are intricately linked, and one has a complex influence on the other. Scientific discoveries have the power to challenge our cultural beliefs and values, just as cultural norms and practices have the power to shape our understanding of science.

10. The scientific endeavor must be sustainable: Lastly, the scientific endeavor must be sustainable in terms of both its financial support and its impact on society and the environment. It is up to us to ensure that scientific research is conducted in a way that benefits society and does not jeopardize the well-being of future generations.

In conclusion, methylene blue has advanced significantly from its modest origins as a laboratory reagent to its present position as a multipurpose instrument in several industries. Because of its special qualities, it is a significant participant in fields including environmental research, biotechnology, and medicine. Methylene blue has a wide range of possible uses, from the detection of water contamination to the treatment of illnesses, if more research and development is conducted. We should expect to see even more creative applications for this potent chemical as technology develops.

Methylene blue has shown a lot of promise in the medical sector for treating some illnesses, such as cancer, malaria, and neurological diseases. It is a compelling substitute for conventional chemotherapy because of its capacity to specifically target and kill cancer cells while sparing healthy cells. Furthermore, its ability to effectively cure malaria has the potential to save many lives, particularly in underdeveloped nations with limited access to healthcare.

Methylene blue has shown promise in environmental research for identifying and eliminating contaminants from water sources. It is a useful instrument for clearing polluted waterways because of its capacity to bind to heavy metals and other dangerous materials. This is especially important given the escalating global water problem and the decreasing availability of safe drinking water.

Moreover, the application of methylene blue in biotechnology has advanced our knowledge of cellular activity and processes. Scientists may investigate the internal workings of cells and learn important information about the mechanisms regulating cellular activity by employing methylene blue as a fluorescent dye. The development of novel therapies and treatments for a variety of illnesses and ailments can then be facilitated by this information.

To sum up, methylene blue has advanced significantly from its humble beginnings as a lab reagent. Its adaptability and efficacy have made it a useful instrument in several domains, with the capacity to enhance human well-being, safeguard the ecosystem, and progress scientific understanding. Methylene blue is a potent chemical, and as a study into its qualities and uses grows, we should anticipate even more significant effects in the years to come.

www.ingramcontent.com/pod-product-compliance
Lightning Source LLC
Chambersburg PA
CBHW070847310526
45796CB00014B/170